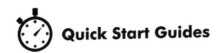 **Quick Start Guides**

G000129512

The Essential
21 DAY SUGAR DETOX
FAT-LOSS PLAN

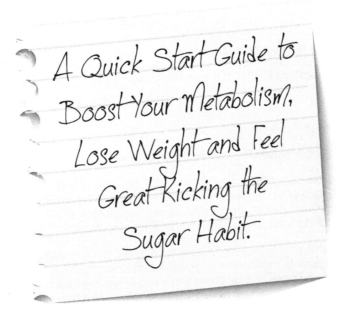

A Quick Start Guide to Boost Your Metabolism, Lose Weight and Feel Great Kicking the Sugar Habit.

No-Fuss, Easy And Delicious Sugar-Free Diet Recipes To Beat Sugar Cravings.

First published in 2018 by Erin Rose Publishing

Text and illustration copyright © 2018 Erin Rose Publishing

Design: Julie Anson

ISBN: 978-1-911492-78-8

A CIP record for this book is available from the British Library.

DISCLAIMER: This book is for informational purposes only and not intended as a substitute for the medical advice, diagnosis or treatment of a physician or qualified healthcare provider. The reader should consult a physician before undertaking a new health care regime and in all matters relating to his/her health, and particularly with respect to any symptoms that may require diagnosis or medical attention.

While every care has been taken in compiling the recipes for this book we cannot accept responsibility for any problems which arise as a result of preparing one of the recipes. The author and publisher disclaim responsibility for any adverse effects that may arise from the use or application of the recipes in this book. Some of the recipes in this book include nuts or other allergens. If you have an allergy it's important to avoid these.

CONTENTS

INTRODUCTION

If you are ready to begin your sugar detox fat-loss plan and kick those sugar cravings for good, now is the time to begin!

No-one ever said ditching the sugar habit was easy but in this easy-to-follow book we provide you with essential advice, tips, recipes and meal plans to make losing weight on a sugar-free diet simple.

Following a sugar free diet is known to reduce belly fat. Excess sugar consumption can cause a sluggish metabolism which becomes insulin resistant as the body tries to process the sugar. So if you have belly fat which is stubborn to shift, kicking the sugar habit is essential for healthy weight loss.

Your metabolism will benefit and you will steadily see your body transforming as those excess pounds disappear. The health benefits of reducing middle fat are huge. Blood sugar issues, cardiovascular disease, and metabolic problems linked with thyroid issues and PCOS all benefit from a sugar free diet. Stress and anxiety are also linked with fluctuations in blood sugar and it's vitally important to balance your sugar levels to feel at your best.

Looking and feeling good starts on the inside. Beginning with how you fuel your body is essential. In this book, our aim is to present what you can eat for fat-loss and better health in a straightforward way.

In this 21-day sugar detox plan you can take control, eat healthily, improve your metabolism and lose weight. Try not to be daunted by the prospect of changing your diet – it's worth it! We provide you with simple steps, delicious recipes and eating plans to make it easy for beginners.

You will enjoy feeling more relaxed, slimmer and healthier. Resetting your body is easier than you think!

Beginning Your Sugar Detox

This book is geared towards detoxing from sugar for 21 days. Some find it beneficial to gradually reduce their sugar consumption to ease into the plan to avoid strong sugar cravings others prefer to cut it out straight away. Bear in mind that cravings are stimulated by eating sugar which activates sensors in the brain to signal to eat even more, so going cold turkey and quitting straight away is preferable. It'll speed up weight loss and end any sugar cravings rather than delay them.

Shorter sugar detox plans may be enticing but the benefits of going sugar-free really kick in after 2 weeks when fat loss is visible and any sugar cravings have died away, by which time you will be enjoying the benefits and finding it easy. The recipes will help stave off cravings without letting you be hungry. After 21 days you may wish to carry on a sugar-free diet, depending on your goals. Everyone loses weight at a different rate and switching to a sugar-free, lower carb diet will affect the metabolism. So to maximise the benefits you can later decide if you wish to repeat the sugar detox plan.

In the meantime, prepare yourself and check out how you may be eating much more sugar than you think. Have a look at the foods to avoid and familiarise yourself with the list so that you're well prepared.

Your cupboards probably contain savoury foods which contain sugars which really add up plus consuming added sugars will cause cravings to some degree so be kind to yourself and avoid them. When it comes to stocking up at the supermarket, always read the label so that you don't sabotage yourself with hidden sugars.

Foods to AVOID

Below is a list of the food categories detailing which foods to REDUCE or AVOID all products containing sugar and starchy carbohydrates. Such as:

- Cakes, muesli, granola, biscuits, cookies, breakfast cereal, cereal bars, syrup, honey, agave, chocolate, jam, sweets and candy. Marinades, dressings and ready-made sauces such as ketchup, sweet chilli sauce, barbecue sauce, and any dressing or processed foods containing sugar.

- Avoid dried fruit, like raisins, apricots, sultanas, mangoes, pineapple, bananas and figs.

- Starchy carbohydrates such as bread, rice cakes, crackers, pasta, potatoes, sweet potatoes, brown and white rice.

- Beware of fruit juices, milk shakes, smoothies, fizzy drinks, cocktails, alcohols and drinks containing sugar and concentrated fruit juice.

- Drinks with artificial sweeteners such as, aspartame, xylitol, sucralose, cyclamates, saccharin, acesulfame potassium.

What You Can Eat:

Eat some protein with every meal. It staves off hunger and has less of an effect on blood sugar. Eat no more than 2 pieces of fruit a day. Low sugar fruit like blueberries, raspberries or blackberries are great.

• Chicken, pork, lamb, turkey and beef.

• Prawns, cod, salmon, tuna, sardines and mackerel – oily fish are especially good.

• Uncoated nuts and seeds such as Brazils, hazelnuts, cashews, peanuts, pecans, sunflower, pumpkin and sesame seeds.

• Dairy products such as cheese, butter and yogurt.

• Eggs.

• Nut butters; peanut, almond, cashew and seeds.

• Eat fresh vegetables in abundance.

• Herbal and fruit teas.

• Beans and pulses such as kidney beans, cannellini beans, black beans, butter beans, chickpeas and lentils.

• Coconut oil, olive oil, avocado oil and vegetable oils.

Simple Steps To Boost Your Metabolism

For those blessed with a fast metabolism, reducing your food intake may be enough to rid yourself of unwanted weight. For many more who seem unable to shed pounds, even after restricting your calorie intake or frequently exercising and being unable to burn off that excess fat – the despair is real!

Apart from factors which are outside our control like genetics, gender, age and height, there are other factors which can affect your metabolism:

- **Hormonal imbalance; thyroid disease, menopause, PMS, fluid retention, diabetes and polycystic ovaries syndrome.**

- **Stress increases cortisol levels, also known as the stress hormone, which slows the metabolism, storing energy to deal with the stress. Chronic stress will see sustained lowering of the metabolic rate.**

- **Some medications like steroids and antidepressants can cause weight gain.**

- **Caffeine and alcohol, although stimulants, can exacerbate stress by increasing adrenaline. Although some say caffeine and alcohol benefit the metabolism, they increase stress which causes your body to store fat.**

- **Irregular eating alerts your body to fear starvation. Starvation mode increases stress which raises cortisol which in turn causes fat to be stored particularly around the middle.**

- **Higher muscle mass requires more energy and burns fat. Therefore less muscle slows your metabolism.**

- **Sleep deprivation causes tiredness and stimulates the appetite to eat more to raise energy levels – often it's the sugary and fatty foods. Stress from lack of sleep may also be a factor.**

What You Can Do

- Not eating enough or eating the majority of your food in one sitting will slow your metabolism. Spreading your food intake throughout the day will gradually fuel your body, preventing fuel storage due to starvation mode kicking in. Eating healthy foods spaced out throughout the day.

- Avoid sugar and refined carbs as they offer a fast injection of fuel which spikes the blood sugar with a quick fix of energy. Far from being a good thing, this intense sugar fix will prevent your body from burning fat stores and slow your metabolism.

- Avoid caffeine and alcohol. If you crave coffee or feel a withdrawal headache coming on, some people can alleviate it by putting a granule or drop under their tongue.

- Green tea contains less caffeine, coming in at 25mg per 8oz whereas a Starbucks coffee has 165mg caffeine per 8oz. If you don't feel stress is an issue you could include green tea in your diet. Research showed the antioxidants in green tea assists the liver in turning fat cells into fuel.

- Reduce stress as much as possible. If you don't get much sleep you may find it improves on the sugar detox so aim to get a good 8 hours sleep a night.

- If you can, try to eat organic where possible. Meat can contain hormone residues which compete with our body to maintain balance between our own hormones.

- Don't eat large meals late at night. Preferably, eat your last meal before 8pm or earlier if you can.

If you have any medical complaints, consult with your doctor to check for any underlying health conditions and also that it's safe for you to embark on a change of diet. Also discuss any changes or concerns about medication.

The Principles Of The Sugar Detox

If you feel daunted at the prospect of starting a sugar detox, rest assured that it gets easier once you get started. Here are the key points to remember!

- **Avoid all products containing sugar or sweeteners.**

- **Lower your carbohydrate intake – it will help balance your blood sugar, metabolism, boost weight loss and reduce sugar cravings.**

- **Never miss a meal. Eat breakfast, lunch and dinner, making sure you have your evening meal before 8pm. You can also eat 1 or 2 healthy snacks a day.**

- **Drink PLENTY of water – at least 4 pints a day. It will not only hydrate you and make you feel fuller, but it will carry away waste products from your organs and aid detoxification. Simple but so necessary to prevent you recycling toxins.**

- **Avoid alcohol and lower your caffeine intake to reduce stimulus and stress on the adrenals.**

Ditch the Hidden Sugars

Always read the labels on everything you buy at the supermarket. You don't want to load up your shopping basket with foods you didn't realise contained sugar. Check out the list of names sugar is also known as and do your best to avoid these.

- Invert sugar syrup
- Cane juice crystals
- Dextrin
- Dextrose
- Glucose
- Glucose syrup
- Sucrose
- Fructose
- Fructose syrup
- Maltodextrin
- Barley malt

- Beet sugar
- Corn syrup
- Date sugar
- Palm sugar
- Malt syrup
- Dehydrated fruit juice
- Fruit juice concentrate
- Carob syrup
- Golden syrup
- Refiners syrup
- Ethylmaltol

Curbing Your Sweet Tooth

Using sweeteners can make you crave the taste of something sweet so try to avoid them. Stevia is a natural sweetener and shows none of the side effects associated with artificial sweeteners.

If you get a sugar craving, eat protein or healthy fats. Consuming fat is satisfying and curbs your appetite instead of fuelling it like sugar does. Be prepared and keep a supply of suitable snacks available; nuts, cubes of cheese, full-fat Greek yogurt, ham or chicken pieces are ideal. Sugar cravings will subside within 3-4 days, so don't give in or you'll prolong them.

Distraction is also helpful. If you've had a meal and have that longing for something sweet do something that takes you away from the kitchen. Take a walk, have a bath or drink a large glass of water or your favourite herbal tea.

Take a look at the recipes and choose something you really like the sound of which you can prepare in advance or that you can have the ingredients handy to rustle up in a hurry.

Comfort eating is a vicious cycle, especially if you reach for chocolate bars, cakes or stodgy white bread, which let's face it, that's what we are drawn to as a mood fixer. Not only does it pile on the pounds but the highs and lows of the blood sugar change can lead to low mood and anxiety and so it begins all over again.

Nuts are a great source of magnesium which is helpful for stress and depression which is going to make life easier all round.

Top Tips For Going Sugar-Free

If sugar cravings kick in well before your next meal, apart from snacking on something high protein one of the best ways to overcome cravings is to use distraction. Literally, get up and do something.

- Snack on protein instead of carbohydrates. Carry on-the-go snacks like nuts, olives, cheese, or cooked meat for quick sustenance.
- At mealtimes, replace starchy carbohydrates with lots of veggies and you'll not only feel less sluggish but less hungry too.
- Drink plenty of water! You could even prepare some cucumber water. Steep sliced cucumber and mint leaves in a large jug of water, store in the fridge and serve with ice and lemon.
- Prepare meals and treats for the fridge or freezer. Have something sugar-free close by so that you aren't tempted.
- Get plenty of rest and sleep.
- High protein foods can help break the cravings for not only sugar but starchy carbohydrates like white bread, biscuits and cakes.
- Start your day with a large glass of water (approx. 1 pint) This may be old news to some but it's is important to hydrate and flush out your system first thing in the morning.
- Don't over-do it with lots of fruit. It does contain fructose which is a form of sugar. You could opt for lower sugar fruits instead. For instance grapes and figs have 16g of sugar per 100g which is high compared to raspberries which contain 4.4g per 100g and rhubarb which has only 1.1g.
- Eating plenty of veggies is not only nutritious it will help fill you up and can substitute carbohydrates.
- If you're finding eating sugar free challenging, or if you fall off the wagon, don't worry. Get straight back onto it and make sure to avoid sugar to subdue any cravings. Keep going. You can do it.
- This book contains recipes for sweet treats. However, if you are struggling you may wish to avoid these for the duration to really beat those cravings. For some, a little of something sweet tasting may be enough so judge for yourself if a little of something will satisfy you or prove too tempting. The same with fruit – it may be best avoided completely to begin with.
- Lastly, NO self-criticism. This isn't about setting yourself impossibly high standards. You've made a wonderful decision to improve your health and every step you take towards optimum health is a great achievement.

21 Day Meal Plan

To get the most out of your 21 day detox, this diet needs to work to fit your individual needs. If following the meal plan doesn't work for you, that's okay. Just make sure you avoid all sugars and lower your carbohydrate intake. There are many recipes included in this book and you can choose what you like – you do not have to follow the meal plans exactly.

The meal plans are an example and for guidance. You can make swaps and substitutions if you wish. Making batches and prepping in advance is a great way to save time and use up leftovers. For instance you can make a batch of soup and use it over 2-3 days or freeze various soups and defrost them as you need. Some prefer to not eat the same meals two days in a row but it may suit you not to waste ingredients and use them up.

We want you to enjoy your food and giving up sugar can be daunting. When you begin your sugar detox there will be a short period of adjustment while your taste buds get used to the change in flavours, especially subtler flavours as sugar is a strong and overwhelming taste.

You can eat snacks such as olives, cubes of cheese, pieces of cooked meat and vegetables. These have not been included in the meal planner as you may not need snacks but don't let yourself become too hungry.

The sweet recipes in this book are to be eaten in moderation only occasionally and remember stimulating your sweet tooth can result in you giving in to further temptation. You could try some of the snack recipes instead and it's a good idea to make them ahead of time to avoid over indulging in readily available unhealthy foods.

Week 1

Day 1	Day 2	Day 3	Day 4	Day 5	Day 6	Day 7
Breakfast	**Breakfast**	**Breakfast**	**Breakfast**	**Breakfast**	**Breakfast**	**Breakfast**
Raspberry yogurt swirl	Blueberry protein pancakes	Pear salad smoothie	Ham & egg mug muffin	Smoked salmon scramble	Blueberry & coconut breakfast bowl	Chocolate proteins shake
Lunch	**Lunch**	**Lunch**	**Lunch**	**Lunch**	**Lunch**	**Lunch**
BLT chicken salad	Carrot and basil soup	Roast red pepper soup	Egg-drop soup	Creamy stuffed tomatoes	Thai chicken Soup	Tuna & chickpea salad
Dinner	**Dinner**	**Dinner**	**Dinner**	**Dinner**	**Dinner**	**Dinner**
Chicken tikka & roast vegetables	Turkey & butter-bean mash	Smoked pork & vegetable skewers	Sea bass & ratatouille	Lamb skewers & yogurt dip	Lemon prawns & Spanish rice	Chicken & avocado wraps

Week 2

Day 1	Day 2	Day 3	Day 4	Day 5	Day 6	Day 7
Breakfast	**Breakfast**	**Breakfast**	**Breakfast**	**Breakfast**	**Breakfast**	**Breakfast**
Parmesan scramble	Creamy berry smoothie	Ginger & lime refresher	Blueberry Protein pancakes	Chocolate & banana smoothie	Ham & egg mug muffin	Raspberry yogurt swirl
Lunch	**Lunch**	**Lunch**	**Lunch**	**Lunch**	**Lunch**	**Lunch**
Spiced Mackerel	Mexican chunky soup	Turkish eggs	Asparagus & poached Egg	Tomato & lentil soup	Feta cheese & butter-bean salad	Cheese & spinach mini omelettes
Dinner	**Dinner**	**Dinner**	**Dinner**	**Dinner**	**Dinner**	**Dinner**
Rosemary chicken & roast vegetables	Tandoori salmon	Chicken fajitas	Lentil curry & cauliflower 'rice'	Halloumi & tomato kebabs	Chickpea & chorizo casserole	Garlic & herb king prawns with Spanish 'rice'

Week 3

Day 1	Day 2	Day 3	Day 4	Day 5	Day 6	Day 7
Breakfast	**Breakfast**	**Breakfast**	**Breakfast**	**Breakfast**	**Breakfast**	**Breakfast**
Kiwi salad smoothie	Smoked salmon scramble	Chocolate protein shake	Strawberry & chia seed breakfast bowl	Blueberry protein pancakes	Creamy berry smoothie	Parmesan scramble
Lunch	**Lunch**	**Lunch**	**Lunch**	**Lunch**	**Lunch**	**Lunch**
Chicken & vegetable soup	Feta cheese & butter-bean salad	Asparagus & poached eggs	Chickpea, lemon & coriander salad	Tomato & lentil Soup	Lentil & bacon soup	Lemon hummus with Celery
Dinner	**Dinner**	**Dinner**	**Dinner**	**Dinner**	**Dinner**	**Dinner**
Chicken cacciatore	Southern pork & beans	Chunky lamb stew	Chicken & avocado wrap	Plaice & roast asparagus	Turkey & chickpea balls	Chinese chicken salad

Recipes

BREAKFAST

Raspberry Yogurt Swirl

Ingredients

100g (3½ oz) plain Greek yogurt

50g (2oz) fresh raspberries

1 tablespoon ground flaxseeds (linseeds)

½ teaspoon ground cinnamon

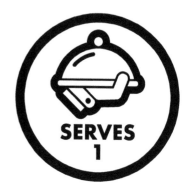

SERVES 1

Method

Place the raspberries into a blender or food processor and blitz to a smooth purée. Place the yogurt into a bowl and mix in the flaxseeds (linseeds) and cinnamon. Add the raspberry purée and partly stir it in leaving swirls in the yogurt. Serve and enjoy.

Blueberry & Coconut Breakfast Bowl

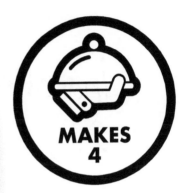

MAKES 4

Ingredients

75g (3oz) blueberries

2 tablespoons chia seeds

1/2 teaspoon vanilla extract

1/2 teaspoon ground cinnamon

100mls (3 1/2 fl oz) coconut milk

100mls (3 1/2 fl oz) milk or almond milk

Method

Place the milk, coconut milk and vanilla extract into a bowl. Add in the chia seeds and stir. Transfer the mixture to 4 dessert glasses or small bowls. Chill the fridge for 1-2 hours and until the mixture has thickened to look like rice pudding. Sprinkle on the cinnamon and scatter the blueberries on top. Enjoy. These delicious little puddings can be stored in the fridge for 2-3 days.

Strawberry & Chia Seed Breakfast Bowl

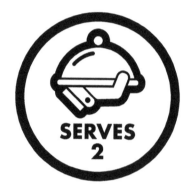

SERVES 2

Ingredients

75g (3oz) strawberries, sliced

2 tablespoons chia seeds

1 teaspoon vanilla extract

200mls (7fl oz) milk or almond milk

Method

Place the chia seeds and almond milk in a bowl and mix well. Cover them and place them in the fridge for 1-2 hours or overnight. In the morning add in the strawberries and vanilla and serve into bowls.

Blueberry Protein Pancakes

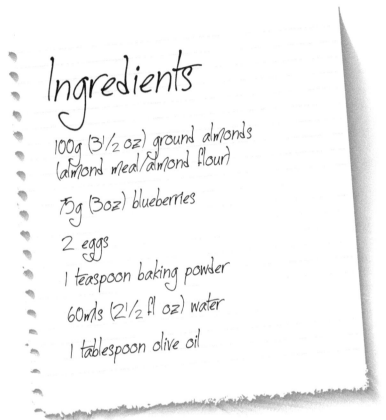

Ingredients

100g (3½ oz) ground almonds (almond meal/almond flour)

75g (3oz) blueberries

2 eggs

1 teaspoon baking powder

60mls (2½ fl oz) water

1 tablespoon olive oil

SERVES 2

Method

Put the eggs in a bowl, whisk them and set aside. Place the almond flour in a bowl and stir in the beaten eggs. Add water and mix until you have a smooth batter. Heat the olive oil in a frying pan. Pour half of the mixture into the pan. Scatter half the blueberries in the pancake mixture and cook until the underside is slightly golden before turning them over to finish cooking. Serve and enjoy.

Chocolate Protein Shake

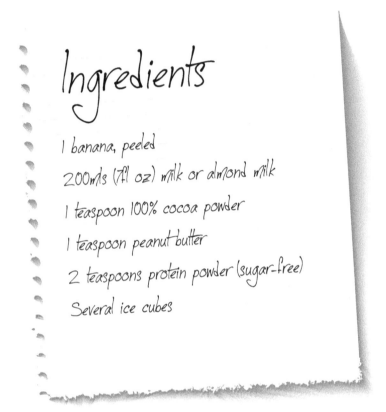

Ingredients

1 banana, peeled

200mls (7fl oz) milk or almond milk

1 teaspoon 100% cocoa powder

1 teaspoon peanut butter

2 teaspoons protein powder (sugar-free)

Several ice cubes

SERVES
1

Method

Place all of the ingredients into blender or food processor and blitz until smooth. Serve into a glass and enjoy!

Kiwi Salad Smoothie

Ingredients

1 kiwi fruit, peeled

1 apple, cored

1/2 small lettuce

Juice of 1/2 lemon

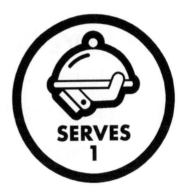

SERVES
1

Method

Place all of the ingredients into a food processor with just enough water to cover them.
Blitz until smooth.

23

Pear Salad Smoothie

Ingredients

1 stalk of celery, roughly chopped

1/2 romaine lettuce, roughly chopped

1 large pear, cored

3 large sprigs of parsley

SERVES
1

Method

Place all of the ingredients into a blender with sufficient water to cover them and blitz until smooth.

Ginger & Lime Refresher

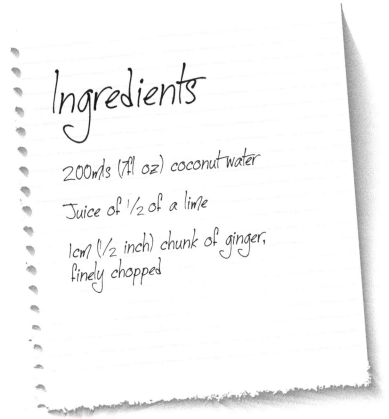

Ingredients

200mls (7fl oz) coconut water

Juice of 1/2 of a lime

1cm (1/2 inch) chunk of ginger, finely chopped

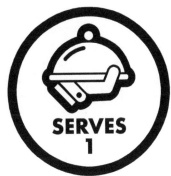

SERVES
1

Method

Mix all of the ingredients in a glass and add a few ice cubes. Drink straight away. This makes a lovely refreshing drink which keeps hunger away.

Chocolate & Banana Smoothie

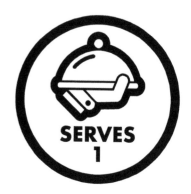

SERVES 1

Ingredients

1 banana

100mls (3½ fl oz) milk or almond milk

1 tablespoon 100% cocoa powder or cacao nibs

1 teaspoon chia seeds

Method

Place all the ingredients into a food processor and mix until smooth and creamy.

Creamy Berry Smoothie

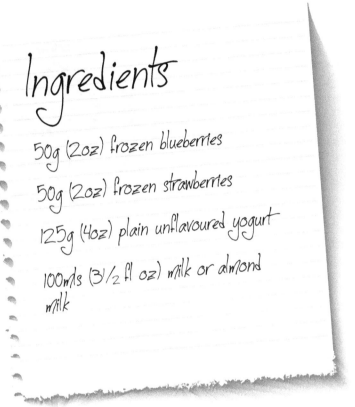

Ingredients

50g (2oz) frozen blueberries

50g (2oz) frozen strawberries

125g (4oz) plain unflavoured yogurt

100mls (3½ fl oz) milk or almond milk

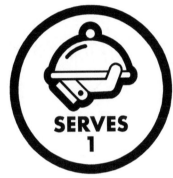

SERVES 1

Method

Whizz the berries, yogurt and milk together in a blender and process until smooth.

Ham & Egg Mug Muffin

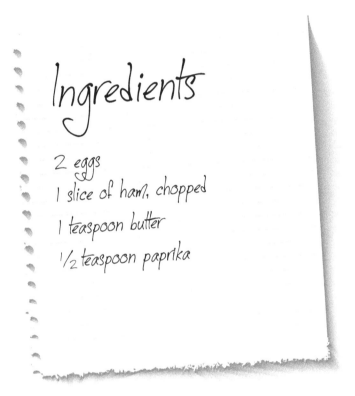

Ingredients

2 eggs
1 slice of ham, chopped
1 teaspoon butter
1/2 teaspoon paprika

**SERVES
1**

Method

Crack the eggs into a large mug and beat them. Add in the butter, ham and paprika and mix well. Place the mug in a microwave and cook on full power for 30 seconds. Stir and return it to the microwave for another 30 seconds, stir and cook for another 30-60 seconds or until the egg is set. Serve it in the mug.

Smoked Salmon Scramble

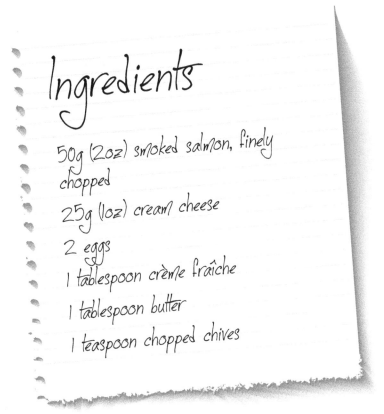

Ingredients

50g (2oz) smoked salmon, finely chopped

25g (1oz) cream cheese

2 eggs

1 tablespoon crème fraîche

1 tablespoon butter

1 teaspoon chopped chives

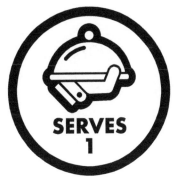

SERVES 1

Method

Crack the eggs into a bowl and whisk in the crème fraîche and chives. Heat the butter in a large frying pan and pour in the egg mixture. Continuously stir and cook the eggs until they begin to set. Stir in the cream cheese and smoked salmon and continue cooking until the eggs have set. Serve and eat immediately.

Parmesan Scramble

Ingredients

2 eggs

1 tablespoon crème fraîche

1 tablespoon grated Parmesan cheese

1 teaspoon fresh oregano, chopped

1 teaspoon fresh basil leaves, chopped

1 teaspoon butter

1/2 teaspoon mixed herbs

SERVES 1

Method

Crack the eggs into a bowl, whisk them up. Add in the Parmesan cheese, crème fraîche, basil, oregano and mixed herbs (if using). Heat the butter in a frying pan. Pour in the egg mixture and stir constantly until the eggs are scrambled and set. Serve and enjoy.

LUNCH

Egg-Drop Soup

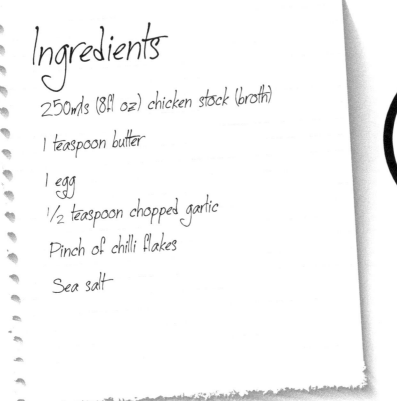

Ingredients

250mls (8fl oz) chicken stock (broth)

1 teaspoon butter

1 egg

1/2 teaspoon chopped garlic

Pinch of chilli flakes

Sea salt

SERVES 1

Method

Heat the butter and chicken stock (broth) in a saucepan and bring it to the boil. Add in the garlic, chilli and salt and stir. Remove it from the heat. In a bowl, whisk the egg then pour it into the saucepan. Stir for around 2 minutes until the egg is cooked. Serve and eat immediately

Carrot & Basil Soup

Ingredients

450g (1lb) carrots, chopped

2 onions, chopped

1 courgette (zucchini), chopped

1 tablespoon olive oil

1200mls (2 pints) hot water

1 handful fresh basil leaves, chopped

SERVES 4

Method

Heat the oil in a saucepan, add the onion and cook for 5 minutes. Add in the carrots and courgette (zucchini) and cook for 5 minutes. Stir in the hot water. Reduce the heat and simmer for 10 minutes. Stir in half of the basil. Using a hand blender or food processor blend the soup until smooth. Re-heat if necessary before serving. Serve with the remaining basil sprinkled over the top.

Lemon Hummus
With Celery

Ingredients

200g (7oz) chickpeas (garbanzo beans), drained

8 stalks of celery

2 cloves of garlic

1 handful fresh basil leaves, roughly chopped

Juice of 1 lemon

1 tablespoon olive oil

1 teaspoon sea salt

**SERVES
4**

Method

Place all of the ingredients, except the celery, into a food processor and process until smooth. Serve as a dip for the celery stalks.

Creamy Stuffed Cherry Tomatoes

Ingredients

125g (4oz) goat's cheese

24 cherry tomatoes, halved

½ teaspoon salt

½ teaspoon freshly ground black pepper

Small handful fresh basil, very finely chopped

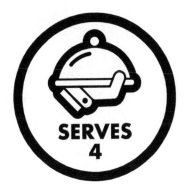

SERVES 4

Method

Place the goat's cheese in a bowl and mix in the chopped basil. Season with salt and black pepper. Gently scoop the tomato seeds and pulp out from inside the tomatoes and pour out any juice. Using a teaspoon scoop some of the mixture into each tomato. Place them on a decorative plate and serve.

Bean & Vegetable Soup

Ingredients

SERVES 4

200g (7oz) frozen soya beans (also called edamame beans)

200g (7oz) frozen peas

50g (2oz) rocket (arugula) leaves

6 spring onions (scallions), trimmed and chopped

1 small bunch basil leaves, chopped

450mls (15fl oz) hot vegetable stock

300mls (½ pint) milk or soya milk

Method

Put the soya beans, peas, vegetable stock (broth) and spring onions (scallions) into a saucepan. Bring it to the boil and simmer for five minutes. Add the basil and rocket (arugula) leaves and soya milk. Pour half of the soup mixture into a food processor and process until smooth. If using a hand blender pour half the soup into a bowl and blitz until creamy. Return the blended soup to the saucepan and warm it through. Serve and enjoy.

Roasted Red Pepper Soup

Ingredients

6 large tomatoes, peeled

4 large red peppers (bell peppers)

4 garlic cloves, unpeeled

1 teaspoon dried oregano

1 red onion, peeled and chopped

900mls (1½ pint) vegetable stock (broth)

Handful of fresh basil leaves

1 tablespoon olive oil

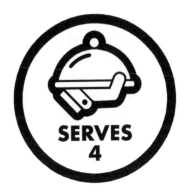

SERVES 4

Method

Place the peppers and garlic on a baking tray, and roast them in the oven at 200C/400F for 30-35 minutes until the skin blisters. Place them in a sealable plastic bag until they cool. Remove them and peel off the skin and throw away the seeds. Heat the olive oil in a large pan, add the onion and cook for 5 minutes until it has softened. Chop the tomatoes and add them to the saucepan along with the peppers (bell peppers), stock (broth), oregano and a few basil leaves. Simmer for 30 minutes. Sprinkle in the basil. Using a hand blender or food processor blitz the soup until smooth. Serve with a garnish of chopped basil leaves.

Pea & Ham Soup

Ingredients

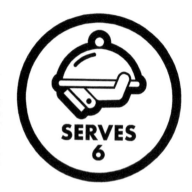

SERVES 6

650g (1lb 7 oz) frozen peas, defrosted

175g (6oz) roast ham or chopped ham hock

1 onion, chopped

3 tablespoons fresh mint, chopped

1 litre (1½ pints) vegetable or chicken stock (broth)

1 tablespoon olive oil

Sea salt

Freshly ground black pepper

Method

Heat the oil in a saucepan, add the onion and cook for 5 minutes until the onion softens. Add in the peas, mint and stock (broth) and cook for 10 minutes. Using a hand blender or food processor blitz the soup until creamy. Stir in the ham and season with salt and pepper. Return it to the heat if necessary. Serve into bowls.

Tomato & Lentil Soup

Ingredients

175g (6oz) red lentils
400g (14oz) tinned chopped tomatoes
2 teaspoons tomato purée
4 tablespoons plain Greek yoghurt
2 celery sticks, chopped
1 onion, peeled and chopped
1 carrot, peeled and chopped
1 garlic clove, crushed
1 teaspoon ground cumin
½ teaspoon ground coriander (cilantro)
1.2 litres vegetable stock (broth)
1 tablespoon olive oil

SERVES
4

Method

Heat the oil in a saucepan and add the onion. Cook for 5 minutes until the onion softens. Add in the celery and carrot and cook for 2 minutes, stirring occasionally. Add the garlic, cumin and coriander and cook for a further minute. Add in the stock (broth), lentils, tomatoes and tomato puree and cook for 20-30 minutes. Using a hand blender or food processor blend the soup until smooth and creamy. Serve into bowls with a swirl of yogurt. Enjoy.

Thai Chicken Soup

Ingredients

SERVES 4

400g (14oz) skinless chicken breast fillets, cut into thin strips

150g (5oz) green beans

6 spring onions (scallions), chopped

1 tablespoon thai curry paste

900mls (1½ pints) chicken stock (broth)

1 tablespoon fish sauce

1 tablespoon olive oil

Juice of ½ lime

Sea salt

Freshly ground black pepper

Handful of fresh coriander (cilantro) leaves, roughly chopped

Method

Heat the oil in a large pan or wok. Add the spring onions (scallions) and cook for 2 minutes. Add in the chicken pieces and cook for 5 minutes. Stir in the Thai curry paste and cook for 1 minute. Pour in the chicken stock (broth) and green beans. Bring to the boil, reduce the heat and simmer for 15 minutes. Squeeze in the lime juice and add the fish sauce. Sprinkle in the coriander (cilantro) and season with salt and pepper. Allow the coriander to wilt for around a minute. Serve into bowls. This is a light soup and coconut milk can be added if desired, by substituting half a pint of the stock for coconut milk.

Lentil & Bacon Soup

Ingredients

400g (14oz) tin chopped tomatoes

200g (7oz) red lentils

6 rashers smoked streaky bacon

2 carrots, peeled and diced

1 onion, peeled and chopped

1.5 litres (2½ pints) vegetable stock (broth)

2 tablespoons chopped fresh parsley

1 tablespoon olive oil

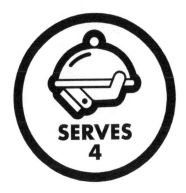

SERVES
4

Method

Heat oil in a large saucepan. Add the bacon, onion and carrots and cook over a medium heat, stirring occasionally, for 8-10 minutes, or until the bacon has started to turn golden and the vegetables have softened. Add the lentils to the pan and stir well. Add the chopped tomatoes and add the stock (broth). Bring to the boil, cover, and then simmer the soup gently for about 1 hour, or until the lentils tender. Allow the soup to cool slightly then using a hand blender or food processor blitz the soup until smooth. Serve into bowls with a sprinkling of parsley.

Mexican Chunky Soup

Ingredients

- 400g (14oz) tin cannellini beans, drained and rinsed
- 200g (7oz) chorizo sausage, sliced
- 3 large carrots, peeled and diced
- 1 onion, peeled and finely chopped
- 1 garlic clove, crushed
- 1 teaspoon chilli powder
- 1 red pepper (bell pepper), deseeded and chopped
- 1 green pepper, deseeded and chopped
- 600mls (1 pint) warm vegetable stock (broth)
- 1 tablespoon olive oil
- Salt and freshly ground black pepper

SERVES 4

Method

Heat the oil in a large saucepan, add the chorizo and cook for 3 minutes. Remove the chorizo and set it aside. Add in the onion, garlic and carrots. Cover and cook gently for about 5 minutes, stirring occasionally. Add in the chilli powder and vegetable stock (broth) and bring to the boil. Return the chorizo to the sauce and add in the peppers (bell peppers) and cannellini beans. Cook for 10-15 minutes. Season with salt and pepper. Serve into bowls.

Turkish Eggs

Ingredients

400g (14oz) tinned chopped tomatoes
2 eggs
1 onion, finely chopped
1 red pepper, finely chopped
1/2 red chilli, finely chopped (more if you like a spicy sauce)
1 clove of garlic, crushed
1/4 teaspoon ground cumin
1/4 teaspoon paprika
1 teaspoon olive oil
Handful of fresh parsley, finely chopped
Sea salt
Freshly ground black pepper

SERVES 1

Method

Heat olive oil in a frying pan. Add the onion, garlic and red pepper and cook for 5 minutes until they soften. Add in the tomatoes, chilli, cumin and paprika. Season with salt and black pepper. Reduce the heat and cook gently for 5 minutes. Crack each of the eggs on top of the tomato mixture and allow them to cook until the eggs are done to your liking. Sprinkle with parsley and serve.

Tuna & Chickpea Salad

Ingredients

SERVES 2

400g (14oz) tin of chickpeas, garbanzo beans

200g (7oz) tin of tuna, drained

75g (3oz) broccoli, broken into florets and halved

75g (3oz) cherry tomatoes

1 red chilli (optional)

1 tablespoon capers

Juice of ½ lemon

Large bunch fresh parsley

Method

Place the broccoli into a steamer and cook for 3 minutes until it has softened. Remove it and allow it to cool. Place the tuna in a bowl and flake it with a fork. Add in the chickpeas (garbanzo beans) and capers and stir well. Add in the tomatoes, parsley and chilli. Once the broccoli has cooled, add it to the ingredients in the bowl. Add in the lemon juice before serving.

Chickpea, Lemon & Coriander Salad

SERVES 2

Ingredients

400g (14oz) tin of chickpeas (garbanzo beans), drained
4 tablespoons fresh coriander (cilantro)
2 spring onions (scallions) finely chopped
1 tablespoon lemon juice
Sea salt
Freshly ground black pepper

Method

Place the chickpeas (garbanzo beans) into a bowl and add in the coriander (cilantro), spring onions (scallions) and lemon juice. Mix the ingredients well. Season with salt and pepper. Eat straight away or store in the fridge until ready to use.

Cheese & Spinach Mini Omelettes

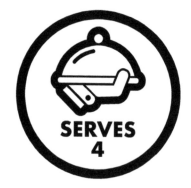

SERVES 4

Ingredients

4 large eggs

50g (2oz) Cheddar, grated (shredded)

75g (3oz) spinach leaves, finely chopped

Method

Place the spinach into a steamer and cook for about 3 minutes until tender. In a bowl, whisk the eggs together then add the cheese. Stir the spinach into the mixture. Lightly grease a 4 portion muffin tin. Pour in the egg and spinach mixture. Bake in the oven at 180C/350F for around 20 minutes until the eggs are set. Enjoy. These can be enjoyed warm or cold.

Chicken & Vegetable Soup

Ingredients

1 whole small chicken

2.5 litres (5 pints) stock (broth)

1 onion, roughly chopped

4 carrots, roughly chopped

4 celery stalks (including leaves) roughly chopped

2 leeks, roughly chopped

1 handful of fresh parsley, chopped

2 sprigs fresh thyme

2 garlic cloves, chopped

SERVES 6

Method

Quarter the chicken into two leg portions and two breast portions and remove any excess fat from the tail and neck. Place all of the chicken in a large saucepan and add the garlic and stock (broth). Bring it to the boil, reduce the heat and simmer for 20 minutes. Using a slotted spoon, skim off any excess grease from the surface of the liquid. Now you can add in the onion, carrots, celery, leeks and thyme. Simmer gently for 1½ hours or until the chicken has completely cooked. Remove the chicken carcass and once again skim off any fat which has floated to the surface. Stir in the chopped parsley. Serve into bowls.

Feta Cheese & Butterbean Salad

SERVES 4

Ingredients

400g (14oz) tin of butter beans

250g (9 oz) cherry tomatoes, halved

125g (4oz) feta cheese, crumbled

75g (3oz) black olives, halved

2 tablespoons fresh basil, chopped

2 tablespoons fresh parsley, chopped

1 cucumber, diced

1 red onion, finely sliced

1 yellow pepper (bell pepper), diced

1 tablespoon olive oil

Juice of ½ lemon

Method

Place the olive oil and lemon juice in a bowl and set aside. Place all of the salad ingredients into a large bowl and mix them together. Pour on the dressing and toss the salad ingredients in the mixture.

Spiced Mackerel

Ingredients

2 mackerel fillets

1 tablespoon fresh coriander (cilantro), chopped

1 red chilli, de-seeded and chopped

1/2 teaspoon ground coriander (cilantro)

1/2 teaspoon ground cumin

Zest and juice of 1 lime

1 teaspoon olive oil

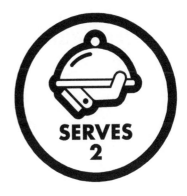

SERVES 2

Method

Place the cumin, fresh and ground coriander (cilantro), chilli, zest and juice of the lime and olive oil in a bowl and mix well. Thickly coat the mackerel with the mixture. Transfer the fish to a hot grill (broiler) and cook for around 4 minutes on each side until cooked through.

Asparagus & Poached Egg

Ingredients

- 150g (5oz) asparagus, tough end removed
- 50g (2oz) green salad leaves
- 1 large egg
- 1 tablespoon olive oil
- 1 tablespoon lemon juice
- Sea salt
- Freshly ground black pepper
- 1 teaspoon parmesan cheese, grated (shredded)
- Dash of vinegar

SERVES 1

Method

Lay the asparagus under a pre-heated grill and cook for 5 minutes on each side. Half fill a saucepan with water and bring it to a simmer. Add in the vinegar and stir. Crack the egg onto a small side plate and slide it into the water. Cook for around 3 minutes until it firms up but remains soft in the middle. Combine the olive oil and lemon juice in a bowl and season it with salt and pepper. Coat the salad leaves with the dressing. Scatter the salad leaves on a plate, serve the asparagus on top and add the egg. Sprinkle with Parmesan cheese and eat straight away.

Eggs With Carrot & Bacon Hash

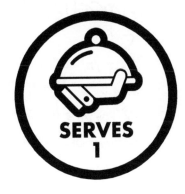

SERVES 1

Ingredients

3 rashers of streaky bacon, finely chopped

2 eggs

1 large carrot, grated

½ onion, finely chopped

1 teaspoon olive oil

Freshly ground black pepper

Method

Heat the oil in a frying pan, add the bacon and onion and cook for 4-5 minutes. Stir in the carrot and cook for 10 minutes. In the meantime, place the eggs into a saucepan of warm water and boil them for 6-7 minutes until the yolks are slightly soft. Season the hash with black pepper and serve it onto plates. Peel and halve the eggs and place them on top of the hash. Eat immediately.

BLT Chicken Salad

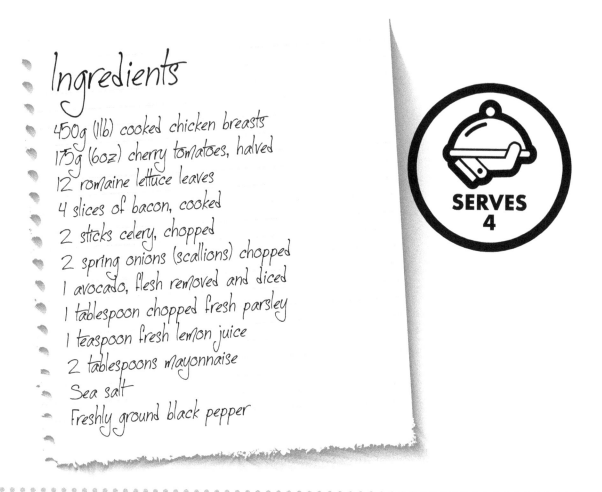

Ingredients

450g (1lb) cooked chicken breasts
175g (6oz) cherry tomatoes, halved
12 romaine lettuce leaves
4 slices of bacon, cooked
2 sticks celery, chopped
2 spring onions (scallions) chopped
1 avocado, flesh removed and diced
1 tablespoon chopped fresh parsley
1 teaspoon fresh lemon juice
2 tablespoons mayonnaise
Sea salt
Freshly ground black pepper

SERVES 4

Method

In a bowl, place the mayonnaise, spring onions (scallions), lemon juice and parsley and mix well. Season with salt and pepper. Add the chicken, bacon, celery and tomatoes to the mixture and stir well. Spoon the mixture into the lettuce leaves and top it off with chunks of avocado. Enjoy.

DINNER

Cauliflower 'Rice'

Ingredients

1 head of cauliflower, broken into florets

2 tablespoons olive oil

Sea salt

Freshly ground black pepper

SERVES 6

Method

Place the cauliflower into a food processor and blitz it until it becomes small rice-like pieces. Heat the oil in a large frying pan and add the cauliflower. Cook for around 5 minutes or until softened. Season and serve. Use it as an alternative to rice, potatoes or pasta as a great accompaniment to meats and salads. It's so easy to jazz up basic cauliflower rice with a teaspoon of paprika or curry powder or mushrooms and chorizo to make a stand alone light meal or to go alongside curries and casseroles.

Spanish 'Rice'

Ingredients

1 head of cauliflower, broken into florets

2 carrots, peeled and roughly chopped

250g (9oz) tomato passata or tinned chopped tomatoes

2 tablespoons olive oil

1 teaspoon chilli powder

1 teaspoon cumin

Small handful of coriander (cilantro)

SERVES 6

Method

Place the cauliflower and carrots into a food processor and blitz until fine and rice-like. Heat the olive oil in a large frying pan, add the cauliflower and carrots and cook for 5-7 minutes or until the vegetables have softened. Add the tomato passata, chilli and cumin and warm it through. Sprinkle in the coriander (cilantro) just before serving.

Lemon Prawns

Ingredients

400g (14oz) cooked frozen prawns, shelled and defrosted

75g (3oz) ground almonds (almond meal/almond flour)

Zest of a lemon, grated (shredded)

1 tablespoon olive oil

Sea salt

White pepper

SERVES 4

Method

Place the ground almonds (almond meal/almond flour) into a bowl. Add in the lemon zest and season with salt and pepper. Add the prawns to the bowl and coat them in the almond mixture. Heat the olive oil in a frying pan. Add the prawns and cook them for around 2 minutes on each side. Serve with a slice of lemon or you can add a dollop of guacamole or mayonnaise. Enjoy.

Smoked Pork & Vegetable Skewers

Ingredients

SERVES 4

400g (14oz) pork steaks, cut into bite-sized chunks

1 tablespoon tomato purée (paste)

1 garlic clove, crushed

1 red pepper (bell pepper), cut into chunks

1 onion, cut into chunks

1 teaspoon smoked paprika

1 tablespoon olive oil

Juice of ½ lemon

Method

Place the paprika, tomato puree (paste) lemon juice, garlic and olive oil into a bowl and mix well. Add the pork pieces to the mixture and coat them thoroughly. Allow them to marinate for at least 1 hour. Thread the marinated pork, red pepper (bell pepper) and onion on skewers, alternating the ingredients. Place the skewers under a pre-heated grill (broiler) and cook for 9-10 minutes, turning during cooking until they are cooked through.

Spiced Citrus & Olive Pork

Ingredients

150g (5oz) pitted green olives
450g (1lb) pork steaks, cut into chunks
2 cloves of garlic, crushed
2 lemons, sliced and seeds removed
1 onion, finely chopped
1 teaspoon ground ginger
1 teaspoon ground coriander
2 teaspoons turmeric
1 tablespoon olive oil
450mls (15fl oz) chicken stock (broth)
Handful of fresh parsley, chopped
Sea salt
Freshly ground black pepper

SERVES 4

Method

Heat the oil in a large saucepan. Add the onion and cook for 5 minutes until it softens. Add the garlic, ginger, coriander (cilantro) and turmeric and cook for 1 minute. Add the pork pieces and cook for 5 minutes, stirring occasionally. Add the sliced lemons and the stock (broth). Season with salt and pepper. Bring it to the boil, reduce the heat and simmer gently for 30 minutes. Add the olives and cook for a further 3 minutes. Stir in the parsley. This dish can be served with salad or cauliflower rice.

Chicken Tikka & Roast Vegetables

Ingredients

SERVES 4

FOR THE CHICKEN:

4 chicken breasts

2.5cm (1 inch) chunk of fresh ginger root, finely chopped

1 clove of garlic, crushed

1 teaspoon chilli powder

1 teaspoon curry powder

1/2 teaspoon sea salt

1/2 teaspoon turmeric

125g (4oz) plain (unflavoured) Greek yogurt

1 tablespoon olive oil

Juice of 1 lemon

FOR THE VEGETABLES:

1 large aubergine (eggplant) cut into thick chunks

4 large tomatoes, de-seeded and cut into chunks

1 red pepper (bell pepper), chopped

1 yellow pepper (bell pepper), chopped

1 tablespoon olive oil

1 handful fresh coriander (cilantro), chopped

Method

For the chicken; place the chilli, salt, curry powder, turmeric, ginger, garlic, yogurt, olive oil and lemon juice into a bowl and stir it well. Coat the chicken in the mixture. Place the vegetables in a large ovenproof dish and coat them in a tablespoon of olive oil. Make a space in the centre of the dish for the chicken breasts or place them on top. Transfer the dish to the oven and cook at 180C/360F for around 35 to 40 minutes or until the chicken is cooked through. Scatter the chopped coriander (cilantro) over the top and serve.

Parmesan & Courgette Bake

SERVES 4

Ingredients

75g (3oz) ground almonds (almond meal/almond flour)

50g (2oz) Parmesan cheese, grated (shredded)

4 tomatoes, evenly sliced

4 courgettes (zucchinis) evenly sliced

1 teaspoon olive oil

Sea salt

Freshly ground black pepper

Method

Grease an ovenproof dish with the olive oil. Place a layer of tomatoes on the bottom of the dish. Now add a layer of courgette (zucchini). Season with salt and pepper. Sprinkle the ground almonds (almond meal/almond flour) over the top. Add a sprinkling of Parmesan cheese. Transfer it to the oven and bake at 180C/360F for 15-20 minutes until the top is golden.

Cheese & Tomato Chicken Breasts

Ingredients

400g (14oz) tinned chopped tomatoes
150g (5oz) cheese, grated
4 chicken breasts
1 teaspoon mixed dried herbs
1 garlic clove, finely chopped
1 onion, chopped
1 red pepper, deseeded and cut into chunks
1 teaspoon tomato purée
1 teaspoon olive oil

SERVES 4

Method

Preheat the oven to 180C/360F. Heat the oil in a frying pan, add the garlic and cook for 2 minutes. Add the chicken and cook for 2 minutes on each side. Transfer the chicken to an ovenproof dish. In a bowl, mix together the tomatoes, tomato purée and herbs. Spread the tomato mixture over the chicken. Transfer it to the oven and cook for 20 minutes. Remove it from the oven and scatter the cheese over the top. Return it to the oven and cook for around 5 minutes or until the chicken is completely cooked and the cheese is bubbling. Serve with vegetables or a heap of salad.

Lamb Skewers & Yogurt Dip

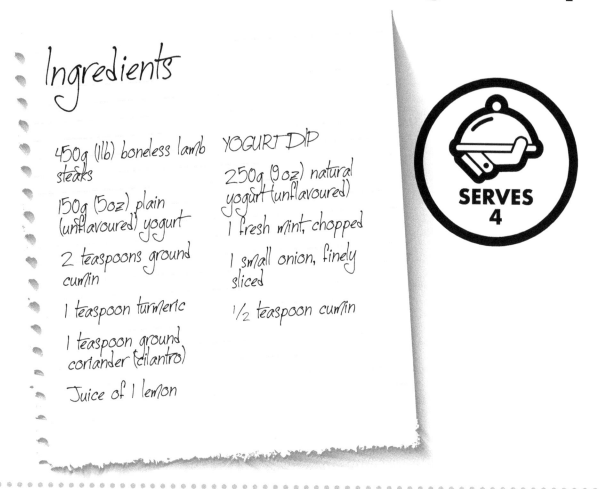

Ingredients

450g (1lb) boneless lamb steaks

150g (5oz) plain (unflavoured) yogurt

2 teaspoons ground cumin

1 teaspoon turmeric

1 teaspoon ground coriander (cilantro)

Juice of 1 lemon

YOGURT DIP

250g (9oz) natural yogurt (unflavoured)

1 fresh mint, chopped

1 small onion, finely sliced

1/2 teaspoon cumin

SERVES
4

Method

Chop the lamb into bite-size chunks. In a bowl, combine the 150g (5oz) yogurt, cumin, turmeric, coriander (cilantro) and lemon juice. Add the lamb to the marinade, cover it and place it in the fridge for one hour. In the meantime, to make the yogurt dip, combine the 250g (9oz) yogurt, chopped onion, mint and cumin. Chill it in the fridge. Once the lamb is marinated, thread the lamb chunks onto skewers. Place under a hot grill (broiler) for 5 minutes on either side. Serve with the dip.

Slow Cooker Vegetable Dahl

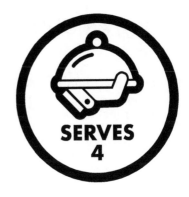

SERVES 4

Ingredients

300g (11oz) yellow split peas

200g (7oz) tinned chopped tomatoes

2 teaspoon ground cumin

2 teaspoon ground turmeric

2 garlic cloves, one crushed, one thinly sliced

2 teaspoons medium curry powder

1 onion, chopped

1 teaspoon ground ginger

1 red chilli, thinly sliced

1 lemon, quartered

600mls (1 pint) hot vegetable stock (broth)

Sea salt

Freshly ground black pepper

Method

Place all of the ingredients into a slow cooker and stir it well. Cook on high for 4 hours until tender. Season with salt and pepper. Serve with a squeeze of lemon on top. This dhal goes well with cauliflower rice as a low carb alternative to your usual white or brown rice.

Quick Bean Chilli

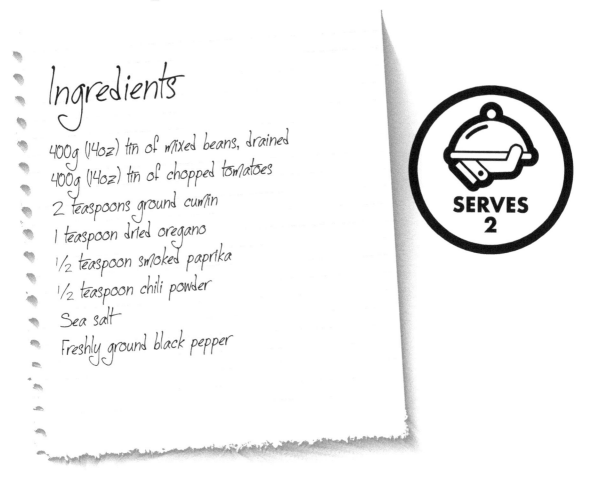

Ingredients

400g (14oz) tin of mixed beans, drained
400g (14oz) tin of chopped tomatoes
2 teaspoons ground cumin
1 teaspoon dried oregano
1/2 teaspoon smoked paprika
1/2 teaspoon chili powder
Sea salt
Freshly ground black pepper

SERVES 2

Method

Place all of your ingredients into a saucepan, bring them to the boil and reduce the heat. Simmer for 10 minutes until the mixture is thoroughly warmed. Serve along with cauliflower rice and green salad.

Mushroom Stroganoff

Ingredients

450g (1lb) closed cup mushrooms, washed and sliced
2 garlic cloves, crushed
1 onion, finely diced
1 teaspoon paprika
1/2 teaspoon English mustard
250mls (9 fl oz) vegetable stock (broth)
200mls (7 fl oz) soured cream
1 tablespoon olive oil
Juice of 1/2 lemon
Sea salt
Freshly ground black pepper

SERVES 4

Method

Heat the oil in a frying pan and add the onion. Cook for 5 minutes until the onion softens. Add the garlic and mushrooms and cook for 5 minutes until the mushrooms are golden. Stir in the paprika and mustard and cook for 1 minute. Pour in the stock (broth) and cook for 5 minutes. Pour in the sour cream and stir well, then add in the lemon juice. Season with salt and pepper. Serve with cauliflower rice.

Sea Bass & Ratatouille

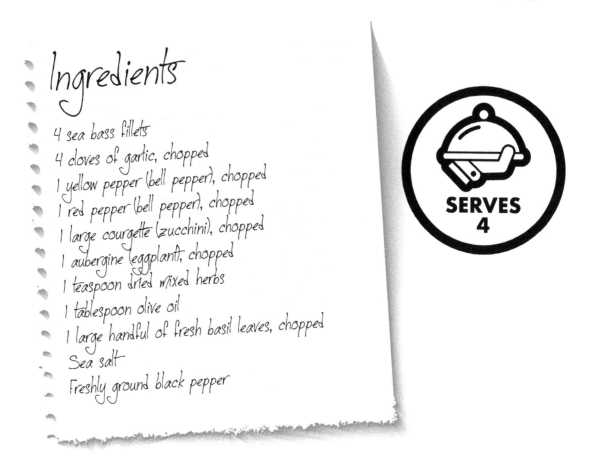

Ingredients

- 4 sea bass fillets
- 4 cloves of garlic, chopped
- 1 yellow pepper (bell pepper), chopped
- 1 red pepper (bell pepper), chopped
- 1 large courgette (zucchini), chopped
- 1 aubergine (eggplant), chopped
- 1 teaspoon dried mixed herbs
- 1 tablespoon olive oil
- 1 large handful of fresh basil leaves, chopped
- Sea salt
- Freshly ground black pepper

SERVES 4

Method

Place the courgette (zucchini) aubergine (eggplant), peppers, garlic, mixed herbs and oil, into an ovenproof roasting dish and toss them well. Season with salt and pepper. Transfer it to the oven and cook at 200C/400F for 25 minutes. Add in half of the fresh basil and stir the vegetables. Place the fish on top of the vegetables. Return it to the oven and cook for 10-12 minutes or until the fish is completely cooked and flakes off. Sprinkle with the remaining basil.

Garlic & Herb King Prawns

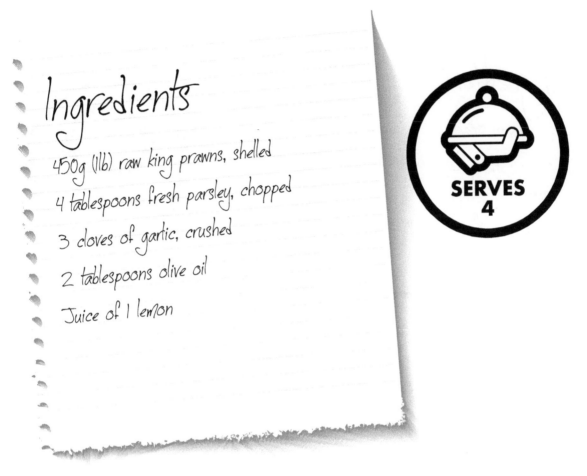

Ingredients

450g (1lb) raw king prawns, shelled

4 tablespoons fresh parsley, chopped

3 cloves of garlic, crushed

2 tablespoons olive oil

Juice of 1 lemon

SERVES 4

Method

In a bowl, place a tablespoon of olive oil, parsley, lemon juice and garlic. Add the prawns and coat them with the mixture. Place in the fridge and marinate for 30 minutes, or longer if possible. When you're ready to cook the prawns, heat a tablespoon of olive oil in a pan. Add the prawns and cook them for around 3-4 minutes until they are cooked through and completely pink. Serve and enjoy.

Tandoori Salmon

Ingredients

- 2 salmon steaks
- 2cm (1 inch) chunk of fresh ginger root, peeled and finely chopped
- 2 cloves of garlic, crushed
- 2 teaspoons paprika
- ½ teaspoon ground cumin
- ½ teaspoon ground coriander (cilantro)
- ¼ teaspoon cayenne pepper (or more to taste)
- 100g (3½ oz) Greek yogurt

SERVES 2

Method

Place all of the ingredients, except the salmon, into a bowl and mix them well. Marinate the salmon in the mixture for at least 1 hour but preferably overnight to allow it to infuse. Place the salmon on a baking tray and cook it in the oven at 200C/400F for 40-45 minutes, or until the salmon is cooked through. Serve with a large green leafy salad.

Turkey & Butterbean Mash

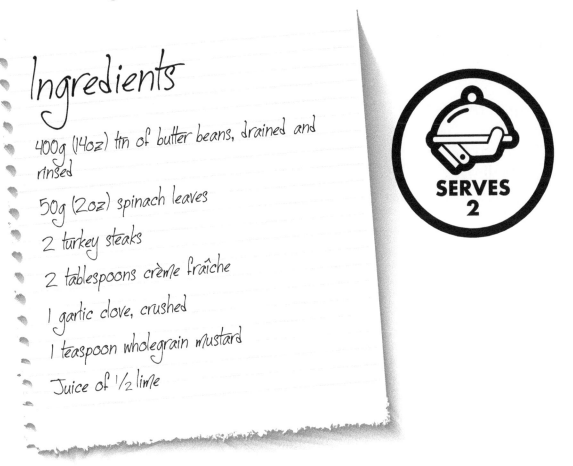

Ingredients

- 400g (14oz) tin of butter beans, drained and rinsed
- 50g (2oz) spinach leaves
- 2 turkey steaks
- 2 tablespoons crème fraîche
- 1 garlic clove, crushed
- 1 teaspoon wholegrain mustard
- Juice of ½ lime

SERVES 2

Method

Place the lime juice and mustard in a bowl and mix together. Add the turkey steaks and coat them well. Place the turkey steaks under a hot grill (broiler) and cook for 5-6 minutes on each side until thoroughly cooked. In the meantime place the butterbeans in a saucepan and add in the garlic and crème fraîche. Season with salt and pepper. Warm the beans thoroughly. Remove the beans from the heat and mash them. Scatter the spinach leaves onto a plate. Spoon the mash on top and add the turkey steaks.

Aubergine & Lentil Bake

Ingredients

- 2 aubergines (eggplants), sliced
- 2 x 400g tins green lentils, drained
- 400g (14oz) tin chopped tomatoes
- 50g (2oz) Cheddar cheese, grated (shredded)
- 2 cloves garlic, sliced
- 2 teaspoon ground cinnamon
- 1 onion, finely chopped
- 1 egg
- 1 carrot finely diced
- 1 tablespoon tomato puree
- Small bunch of oregano, chopped
- 300mls (½ pint) plain (unflavoured) yogurt
- 200mls (7fl oz) vegetable stock (broth)
- 1 tablespoon lemon juice
- 1 tablespoon olive oil
- 1 bay leaf

SERVES 4

Method

Heat the oil in a frying pan, add the onions and garlic and cook for 4 minutes until softened. Add the lentils, carrots, stock (broth) tomatoes and tomato purée, oregano, cinnamon, lemon juice and bay leaf. Bring it to the boil, reduce the heat and simmer for 30 minutes. In the meantime place the aubergine slices under a preheated grill (broiler) and cook on both sides until slightly golden. In a bowl, combine the yogurt, Parmesan cheese and egg. When the lentil mixture has completely cooked, spoon half of the mixture into an ovenproof lasagne dish and place a layer of aubergine (eggplant) on top. Add a second layer of the lentil mixture and add another layer of aubergine. Spread the yogurt mixture on top. Sprinkle with grated cheese. Transfer it to the oven and bake at 180C/360F for 45 minutes and cook until golden.

Rosemary Chicken & Roast Vegetables

Ingredients

SERVES 4

- 250g (9oz) cherry tomatoes, halved
- 4 chicken breasts
- 1 aubergine (eggplant), roughly chopped
- 2 courgettes (zucchinis), roughly chopped
- 2 red peppers (bell peppers), sliced
- 1 green pepper (bell pepper), sliced
- 4 sprigs of fresh rosemary
- 2 cloves of garlic, chopped
- 2 tablespoon olive oil

Method

In a large ovenproof dish, spread the aubergine (eggplant), courgettes, (zucchinis) and peppers (bell peppers) with 2 sprigs of rosemary, 1 clove of garlic and a tablespoon of olive oil. Transfer it to the oven and cook at 200C/400F for 20 minutes. In the meantime, mix the remaining garlic, rosemary and olive oil in a bowl. Make an incision in the chicken breasts and spread some of the mixture into each one. Once the vegetables have been in for 20 minutes, add the tomatoes and chicken breasts to the dish. Return it to the oven and cook for another 20 minutes and cook until the chicken is thoroughly cooked.

Moroccan Tuna Steaks

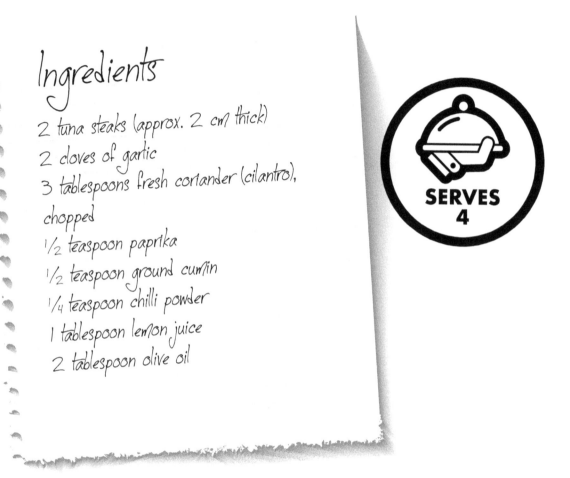

Ingredients

2 tuna steaks (approx. 2 cm thick)
2 cloves of garlic
3 tablespoons fresh coriander (cilantro), chopped
1/2 teaspoon paprika
1/2 teaspoon ground cumin
1/4 teaspoon chilli powder
1 tablespoon lemon juice
2 tablespoon olive oil

SERVES 4

Method

Place the olive oil, garlic, coriander (cilantro), paprika, cumin, chilli powder and lemon juice into a food processor and blitz until smooth. Transfer the mixture to a bowl and place the tuna steaks in the marinade. Allow it to sit for 30 minutes. Heat a frying pan and add the tuna steaks. Cook for 3-6 minutes, depending on how well done you like them cooked, turning once in between. Serve and eat straight away.

Turkey & Chickpea Balls

Ingredients

400g (14oz) tin of chickpeas (garbanzo beans), rinsed and drained

250g (9oz) turkey mince (ground turkey)

50g (2oz) chickpea flour (garbanzo bean flour/gram flour)

2 tablespoons olive oil

2 garlic cloves, finely chopped

1 teaspoon cumin

1/2 onion, chopped

1/2 teaspoon baking powder

Sea salt

Freshly ground black pepper

SERVES 4

Method

Place all of the ingredients into a food processor and mix until everything is chopped and well combined. Transfer the mixture to a bowl, cover it and chill in the fridge for around 30 minutes for the mixture to firm slightly. Take a spoonful of the mixture, and using wet hands, shape it into a ball shape. Heat the olive oil in a frying pan, add the balls and cook them for 12-15 minutes, turning frequently until cooked through. Serve with guacamole or mayonnaise and salad.

Chicken Cacciatore

Ingredients

250g (9 oz) mushrooms, sliced

4 chicken breasts

2 x 400g (14oz) tins of chopped tomatoes

2 green peppers (bell peppers) chopped

1 onion, finely diced

1 tablespoon tomato paste (purée)

1 teaspoon dried basil

2 cloves garlic, chopped

SERVES 4

Method

Place all ingredients in the slow cooker and stir them well. Place the lid on the slow cooker and cook for 6-7 hours. Serve with mashed cauliflower, salad or roast vegetables.

Chicken Fajitas

Ingredients

FOR THE SALSA:

1 red onion, finely chopped

400g (14oz) tomatoes, chopped

2 garlic cloves, crushed

A large handful of fresh coriander leaves, chopped

Freshly ground black pepper

FOR THE CHICKEN FAJITAS

4 large chicken breasts, cut into strips

1 red onion, thinly sliced

1 red pepper (bell pepper) thinly sliced

1 yellow pepper (bell pepper) thinly sliced

1 large romaine lettuce, separated into leaves

1/2 teaspoon paprika

1/2 teaspoon mild chilli powder

1/2 teaspoon ground cumin

1/2 teaspoon dried oregano

1 tablespoon olive oil

SERVES 4

Method

FOR THE SALSA:
Place all the ingredients for the salsa into a bowl and combine them. Season with pepper. Chill in the fridge for 20 minutes.

FOR THE FAJITAS:
Heat the olive oil in a large frying pan, add the onion and peppers. Cook for 3 minutes until the vegetables begin to soften. Add in the chicken, paprika, cumin, chilli powder and oregano and stir well. Cook for around 6 minutes, or until the chicken is thoroughly cooked. Serve the chicken mixture inside a lettuce leaves and add a spoonful of salsa on top. Enjoy. You could also add guacamole or sour cream to your fajita.

Fish Casserole

Ingredients

- 250g (9oz) frozen cooked prawns, peeled
- 150g (5oz) fresh scallops
- 100g (3 1/2oz) mushrooms
- 2 x 400g (2 x 14oz) tins chopped tomatoes
- 2 cloves garlic, finely chopped
- 1 onion, finely chopped
- 1 red pepper, chopped
- 1 green pepper, chopped
- 1 bay leaf
- 1 tablespoon fresh parsley, chopped
- 1/2 teaspoon ground cumin
- 1/2 teaspoon cayenne pepper
- 200mls (7fl oz) chicken stock (broth)
- 1 tablespoon olive oil
- Sea salt
- Freshly ground black pepper

SERVES 4

Method

Heat the olive oil in a large saucepan. Add the onions and cook for 4 minutes until the onion softens. Add in the mushrooms, peppers (bell peppers) and garlic. Cook for 10 minutes, stirring occasionally. Add in the stock (broth) cumin, cayenne, tomatoes, bay leaf, salt and pepper. Bring it to the boil, reduce the heat and simmer for 30 minutes. Add in the scallops and prawns and cook for 15 minutes. Remove the bay leaf before serving the casserole. Season with salt and pepper and serve with a sprinkling of parsley.

Parsley & Lemon Salmon

Ingredients

50g (2oz) spinach leaves

2 salmon fillets

2 tablespoons fresh parsley, chopped

2 tablespoons olive oil

1 clove of garlic

Juice of 1 lemon

Freshly ground black pepper

SERVES 2

Method

Mix together the lemon juice, 2 tablespoons olive oil, garlic and parsley and season with pepper. Place the fish on a plate and lightly coat each fillet with the lemon & parsley mixture. Heat a frying pan and add the salmon. Cook for 3-4 minutes on each side and check that it's completely cooked. Scatter the spinach leaves onto plates. Serve the fish on top and spoon over the remaining lemon and parsley dressing. Enjoy.

Chinese Chicken Salad

Ingredients

FOR THE DRESSING:

2 tablespoons tahini paste (sesame seed paste)

1 clove of garlic, finely chopped

1 tablespoon soy sauce

2 tablespoons fresh lemon juice

Sea salt

Freshly ground black pepper

FOR THE SALAD:

2 skinless chicken breasts, cooked

12 cm (5 in) piece cucumber, cut into fine strips

2 carrots, cut into fine strips

1 red pepper (bell pepper), cut into fine strips

2 Little Gem lettuces, separated into leaves

Small handful of fresh basil leaves, finely shredded

Small handful of fresh mint leaves, finely shredded

8 spring onions, halved lengthways

125g (4oz) button mushrooms, finely sliced

SERVES 2

Method

Place the tahini (sesame seed paste), garlic, soy sauce and lemon juice into a bowl and mix well. Season with salt and pepper. Arrange the salad ingredients onto a serving plate and sprinkle the fresh herbs over the top. Scatter over the shredded basil and mint. Cut the chicken into strips and scatter it on top. Pour the dressing into a small bowl and serve.

Chicken, Cannellini & Almond Bake

Ingredients

450g (1lb) chicken thighs, skin removed

400g (14oz) tin of cannellini beans

50g (2oz) almonds, roughly chopped

2 onions, cut into quarters

2 red peppers, (bell peppers), sliced

2 garlic cloves, finely chopped

1 teaspoon ground cumin

1 teaspoon smoked paprika

2 tablespoons olive oil

Juice and zest of 1 lemon

SERVES 4

Method

Place the chicken in a large bowl along with the cannellini beans, onion and peppers. In a separate bowl, place the garlic, cumin, paprika, olive oil and lemon zest and juice. Mix it well, then scoop the mixture into the bowl with the chicken and coat everything with the dressing. Transfer it to a large oven-proof dish and cook in the oven at 180C/ 360F for 45 minutes. Sprinkle in the almonds and cook for another 5 minutes. Serve and enjoy.

Lentil Curry

Ingredients

125g (4oz) green lentils
100g (3½ oz) spinach leaves
25g (1oz) fresh coriander (cilantro) chopped
2 cloves of garlic, chopped
1 onion, chopped
1 red chilli, finely chopped
1 carrot, chopped
1 tablespoon tomato purée (tomato paste)
1-2 teaspoons curry powder
200mls (7fl oz) coconut milk
360mls (12fl oz) vegetable stock (broth)
1 teaspoon coconut oil

SERVES
2

Method

Heat the coconut oil in a frying pan and add the carrot and onion. Cook for 5 minutes until the vegetables have softened. Add the chilli and garlic and cook for 1 minute. Stir in the lentils, tomato puree and the curry powder. Cover and cook for 2 minutes. Pour in the coconut milk and the vegetable stock (broth), bring it to the boil then reduce the heat and cover it. Simmer for 30 minutes. Add in the spinach and stir until it has wilted. Sprinkle in the coriander (cilantro) and enjoy.

Plaice & Roast Asparagus

Ingredients

- 300g (11oz) tender-stem broccoli
- 4 plaice fillets
- 3 cloves of garlic, chopped
- 2 large handfuls of fresh herbs (oregano, parsley or basil)
- 1 large bunch of asparagus
- 1 lemon, cut into wedges
- 1 teaspoon lemon zest
- 2 tablespoons olive oil
- Sea salt
- Freshly ground black pepper

SERVES
4

Method

Preheat the oven to 180C/360F. Pour a tablespoon of olive oil into a roasting tin. Add the garlic, broccoli and asparagus and toss it in the oil. Lay the fish on top of the vegetables. Drizzle a tablespoon of olive oil over the fish and vegetables. Sprinkle on the half of the chopped herbs, lemon zest and season with salt and pepper. Transfer it to oven and cook for around 15 minutes, or until the fish is completely cooked. Toss the remaining herbs over the top and serve with a wedge of lemon.

Chicken & Avocado Wraps

Ingredients

50g (2oz) soya beans

1 cooked chicken breast, finely chopped

½ cucumber, peeled, deseeded and chopped

Flesh of ½ avocado

Juice ½ lemon

1 teaspoon olive oil

4 little gem lettuce leaves

SERVES 1

Method

Place the soya beans in hot water and cook for 2-3 minutes. Rinse them in cold water and set aside. Place the avocado, olive oil and lemon juice in a food processor and mix until smooth and creamy. Put the chicken, beans and cucumber in a bowl and add the avocado mixture. Stir it well to combine it. Scoop some of the mixture into each of the lettuce leaves. Eat straight away.

Pine Nut & Avocado Courgetti

Ingredients

2 medium courgettes (zucchinis)

2 teaspoons pine nuts

1 avocado, stone and skin removed

Juice of 1 lemon

1 teaspoon olive oil

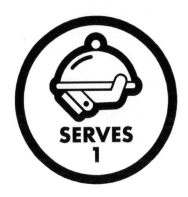

SERVES 1

Method

Use a spiraliser to spiral the courgette (zucchini) into spaghetti lengths. If you don't have a spiraliser, finely slice the courgette into long strips then set them aside. Heat the oil in a frying pan, add the courgette (zucchini) and cook for 5 minutes or until softened. In the meantime, place the avocado, lemon juice and olive oil in a blender and process until it becomes creamy. When the courgette is cooked, spoon the avocado mixture through the courgette and toss in the pine nuts. Serve and enjoy.

Herby Roast Vegetables

Ingredients

150g (5oz) cherry tomatoes, halved

150g (5oz) button mushrooms

3 celery stalks, chopped

3 cloves of garlic, peeled and chopped

2 carrots, peeled and roughly chopped

1 whole beetroot, washed and roughly chopped

1 large onion, chopped

1 courgette (zucchini), chopped

1 butternut squash, peeled and cut into chunks

1 teaspoon dried thyme

1 teaspoon dried oregano

1 large handful of fresh parsley

1 tablespoon olive oil

Sea salt

Freshly ground black pepper

SERVES 4

Method

Place all of the vegetables into an ovenproof dish. Sprinkle in the dried herbs, garlic and olive oil and toss all of the ingredients together. Season with salt and pepper. Transfer them to an oven, preheated to 180C/360F and cook for 30-40 minutes or until all of the vegetables are softened. Scatter in the fresh parsley just before serving.

Chunky Lamb Stew

Ingredients

450g (1lb) lamb steaks, cubed

2 x 400g (14oz) tin of butterbeans

2 carrots, coarsely chopped

2 leeks

1 onion, coarsely chopped

1 teaspoon dried rosemary

400mls (14fl oz) vegetable stock (broth)

1 tablespoon olive oil

SERVES 4

Method

Heat the oil in a saucepan and add in the lamb. Cook for 5 minutes then stir in the carrots, onion and leeks. Cook for a further 5 minutes. Add in the vegetable stock and rosemary. Cover the saucepan and cook on a low heat for around 1 hour. Add in the butterbeans and cook for another 20 minutes. Serve and enjoy.

Halloumi & Tomato Kebabs

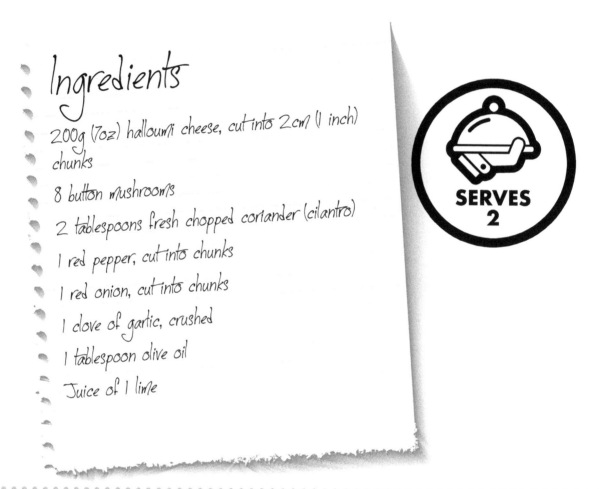

Ingredients

200g (7oz) halloumi cheese, cut into 2cm (1 inch) chunks

8 button mushrooms

2 tablespoons fresh chopped coriander (cilantro)

1 red pepper, cut into chunks

1 red onion, cut into chunks

1 clove of garlic, crushed

1 tablespoon olive oil

Juice of 1 lime

SERVES 2

Method

Place the olive oil, coriander (cilantro), garlic and lime into a bowl and mix well. Season with black pepper. Add the halloumi, mushrooms, onion and red pepper (bell pepper) and allow it to marinate for around 1 hour. Thread the ingredients onto skewers alternating them until everything has been used up. Place the kebabs under a preheated grill (broiler) for 10-12 minutes, turning once halfway through. Serve with a green leafy salad.

Chickpea & Chorizo Casserole

Ingredients

450g (1lb) skinless chicken thighs

400g (14oz) tin of chopped tomatoes

225g (8oz) chickpeas, drained

100g (3½ oz) chorizo, cut into bite-sized chunks

3 cloves garlic, chopped

2 red peppers (bell peppers), chopped

2 teaspoon ground coriander (cilantro)

1 onion, chopped

200mls (7fl oz) chicken stock (broth)

1 tablespoon olive oil

Sea salt

Freshly ground black pepper

SERVES
4

Method

Heat the oil in a frying pan, add the chicken thighs and cook until golden. Remove them from the pan and set aside. Add the chorizo to the oil and cook for 2 minutes. Add in the onions, garlic, red peppers (bell peppers) and coriander (cilantro) and cook for 3 minutes. Pour in the chopped tomatoes, chickpeas (garbanzo beans) and the stock (broth) and add the chicken thighs. Bring it to the boil and simmer for 25 minutes. Season with salt and pepper. Serve with roast vegetables.

Southern Pork & Beans

Ingredients

- 400g (14oz) tin chopped tomatoes
- 2 x 400g (14oz) tins cannellini beans, drained
- 250g (9oz) pork tenderloin fillet, diced
- 150g (5oz) gammon steak, diced
- 2 tablespoons tomato purée
- 2 teaspoons English mustard
- 2cm (1 inch) chunk of ginger, finely chopped
- 2 garlic cloves, finely chopped
- 2 teaspoons smoked paprika
- 1 small handful of parsley, chopped
- 1 onion, sliced
- 1/2 teaspoon hot chilli powder
- 4 tablespoons plain yogurt
- 400mls (14fl oz) chicken stock (broth)
- 1 tablespoon olive oil
- Sea salt
- Freshly ground black pepper

SERVES 4

235 calories per serving

Method

Heat the olive oil in a large frying pan, add the onion and cook for 4 minutes. Stir in the pork and gammon and cook for 3 minutes. Add the garlic, ginger, paprika and chilli powder and cook for 30 seconds or so before adding in the tomatoes and beans. Mix really well. Add in the tomato purée and mustard. Pour over the stock (broth) and simmer for 25 minutes, stirring occasionally, until the pork is completely cooked and tender. Stir in the yogurt and half of the parsley. Season with salt and pepper. Serve with an extra sprinkling of parsley.

SUGAR-FREE DESSERT & SWEET TREAT RECIPES

Macadamia & Coconut Bites

Ingredients

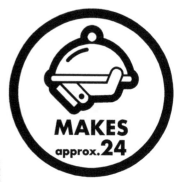

MAKES approx. **24**

- 125g (4oz) almond butter
- 75g (3oz) desiccated (shredded) coconut
- 75g (3oz) macadamia nuts, chopped
- 2 tablespoons tahini paste
- 1 teaspoon stevia sweetener (or more to taste)
- Extra coconut for rolling

Method

Place the coconut, tahini, almond butter and chopped macadamia nuts into a bowl and combine them thoroughly. Stir in a teaspoon of stevia powder then taste to check the sweetness. Add a little more sweetener if you wish. Roll the mixture into balls. Scatter some desiccated (shredded) coconut on a plate and coat the balls in it. Keep them refrigerated until ready to use.

Macaroons

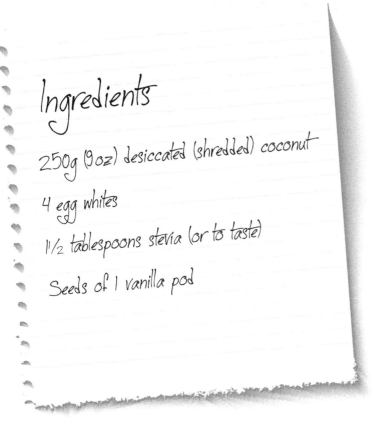

Ingredients

250g (9oz) desiccated (shredded) coconut

4 egg whites

1½ tablespoons stevia (or to taste)

Seeds of 1 vanilla pod

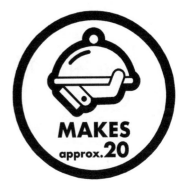

MAKES approx.**20**

Method

Whisk the eggs in a large bowl, until they form stiff peaks. Add in the vanilla and coconut and combine all of the ingredients. Line a baking sheet with parchment paper. Use a teaspoon and scoop out some mixture, rolling it into a small ball then gently flatten it. Place it on the baking sheet and repeat for the remaining mixture. Transfer it to the oven and bake at 180C/360F for around 12 minutes or until the macaroons are golden.

Rhubarb & Ginger Compote With Greek Yogurt

SERVES 2

Ingredients

200g (7oz) plain Greek yogurt

4 stalks of rhubarb, leaves removed and roughly chopped

2cm (1inch) chunk of fresh root ginger, peeled

Zest and juice of 1 orange

¼ teaspoon of stevia or to taste (optional)

Method

Place the rhubarb chunks in a saucepan and add in the zest and juice of the orange together with the ginger and stevia (if using). Warm it gently until the rhubarb becomes soft and pulpy. Remove it from the heat and allow it to cool. Serve the yogurt into decorative bowls and serve the rhubarb compote on top.

Peanut Butter Frozen Yogurt

Ingredients

450g (1lb) plain (unflavoured) yogurt
120mls (4fl oz) milk or non-dairy milk
125g (4oz) smooth peanut butter
1 teaspoon vanilla extract
1/4 teaspoon salt
1-2 tablespoons stevia (to taste)

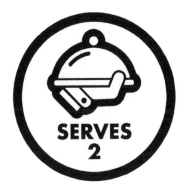

SERVES 2

Method

Place all of the ingredients into an ice-cream maker and mix according to the instructions for your machine. If you don't have an ice-cream maker, transfer the mixture to a container and place it in the freezer and stir the mixture ever ½ hour or so until it becomes firm. As an alternative you can add dark chocolate chips to your frozen yogurt. Delicious!

Chocolate Chip Peanut Butter Cookies

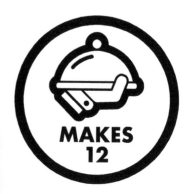

MAKES 12

Ingredients

175g (6oz) peanut butter

25g (1oz) dark chocolate chips (min 75% cocoa)

25g (1oz) walnuts, chopped

25g (1oz) ground flaxseeds

1 large egg

1 teaspoon vanilla extract or seeds of 1 vanilla pod

Method

Place all of the ingredients into a mixing bowl and combine them. Grease and line a baking sheet with parchment paper. Scoop out a spoonful of the mixture and place the mixture on it, flattening it with the back of a spoon. Repeat for the remaining mixture. Transfer it to the oven and bake at 180C/360F for 15-18 minutes or until golden.

Raspberry Panna Cotta

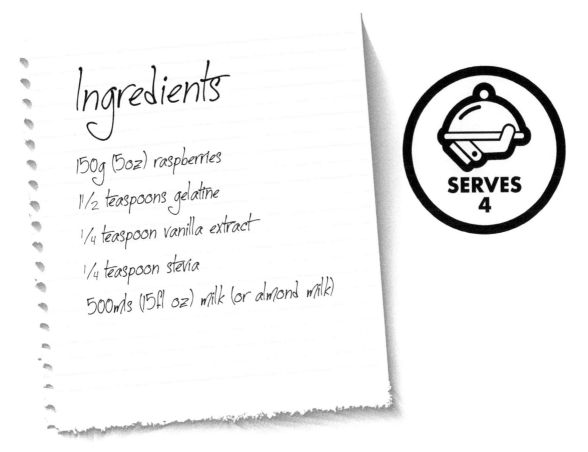

Ingredients

150g (5oz) raspberries

1½ teaspoons gelatine

¼ teaspoon vanilla extract

¼ teaspoon stevia

500mls (15fl oz) milk (or almond milk)

SERVES 4

Method

Pour the almond milk into a bowl and add the gelatine. Allow it to stand for 2-3 minutes until it swells. Pour the almond milk into a saucepan and stir it constantly whilst bringing it to a simmer. Stir in the stevia and vanilla and remove it from the heat. Allow it to cool. In the meantime place the raspberries in the ramekin dishes. Once the mixture has cooled, pour the almond milk mixture into the ramekin dishes. Place the dishes in the fridge for 3-4 hours to set.

SAVOURY SNACK RECIPES

Spiced Bean Balls

Ingredients

150g (5oz) broad beans, soaked in water overnight

1 onion, chopped

1 garlic clove, crushed

1 red chilli, chopped

2 teaspoons ground cumin

1 teaspoon olive oil

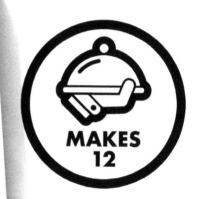

MAKES 12

Method

Place all of the ingredients into a food processor and blend to a smooth paste. Shape the mixture into balls and place them on a greased baking tray. Transfer them to the oven and bake at 180/360F for 20 minutes.

Cashew Crust Kale Chips

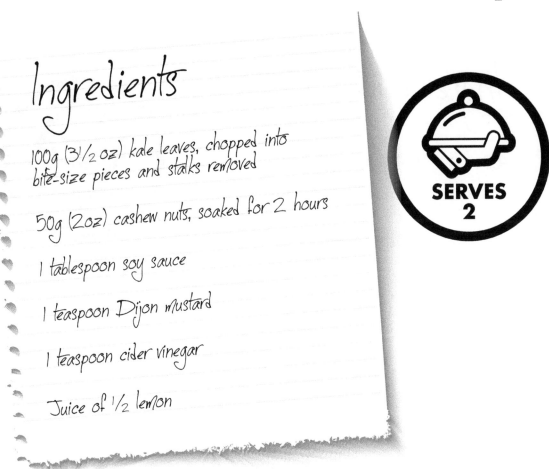

Ingredients

100g (3½ oz) kale leaves, chopped into bite-size pieces and stalks removed

50g (2oz) cashew nuts, soaked for 2 hours

1 tablespoon soy sauce

1 teaspoon Dijon mustard

1 teaspoon cider vinegar

Juice of ½ lemon

SERVES 2

Method

Place the cashews, lemon juice, soy sauce, mustard and vinegar into a food processor and blitz until smooth. Spread the cashew mixture onto the kale, coating it well. Scatter the kale leaves on a large baking sheet. Transfer them to the oven and bake at 180C/360F for 12-15 minutes until slightly golden. Allow them to cool before serving.

Spicy Roast Chickpeas

Ingredients

400g (14oz) tin chickpeas (garbanzo beans), drained

1/4 teaspoon cayenne pepper

1 tablespoon olive oil

Sea salt

SERVES
2

Method

Place the olive oil, salt and cayenne pepper into a bowl and stir well. Add the chickpeas to the bowl and coat them in the olive oil mixture. Spread the chickpeas on a baking sheet. Transfer them to the oven and bake at 220C/ 425F and cook for 30 minutes or until golden. Enjoy as an anytime snack.

Avocado Fries

Ingredients

25g (1oz) ground almonds (almond meal/almond flour)

1 avocado

1 egg

1/2 teaspoon onion powder

1/4 teaspoon chilli powder

1/4 teaspoon sea salt

1 teaspoon water

1 teaspoon olive oil

SERVES
1

Method

Halve the avocado and remove the stone and the skin. Cut it into slices of around 1-2cms thick. Whisk the egg in a bowl and set aside. Place the ground almonds (almond meal/almond flour) into a bowl and add the onion powder, chilli, water and salt. Dip the avocado slices in the beaten egg and then dip it in the almond mixture, coating it well. Coat a baking sheet with olive oil and lay the avocado slices on it. Transfer it to the oven and cook for 15-20 minutes at 180C/360F, turning the slices half way through and cooking until slightly golden. Serve and eat straight away.

Curried Pumpkin Seeds

Ingredients

300g (11oz) pumpkin seeds

1/2 teaspoon sea salt

1/2 teaspoon mild curry powder

1 tablespoon olive oil

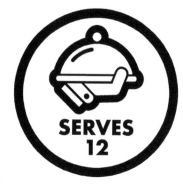

SERVES 12

Method

Place the olive oil, curry powder and salt into a bowl and stir well. Add the pumpkin seeds to the bowl and coat them in the mixture. Scatter the pumpkin seeds on a baking sheet. Transfer them to the oven and bake at 140C/ 280F for 15 minutes. Remove them from the oven and allow them to cool. Enjoy.

Basil & Tomato Olives

Ingredients

50g (2oz) pitted green olives

1 tablespoon fresh basil, chopped

1 tomato, chopped

1 cloves of garlic chopped

Black pepper

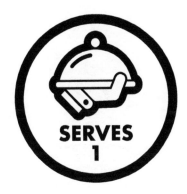

SERVES 1

Method

Place all of the ingredients into a bowl and mix well. Chill before serving.

You may also be interested in other titles by
Erin Rose Publishing
which are available in both paperback and ebook.

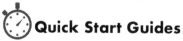 Quick Start Guides

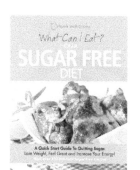
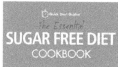
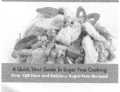
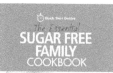
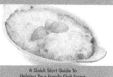
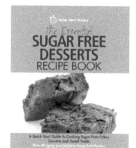
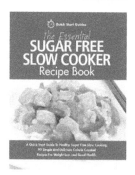
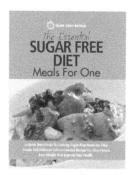
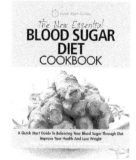
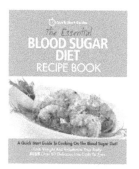
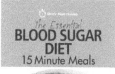
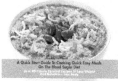
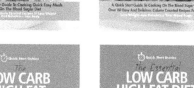
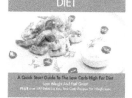
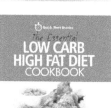
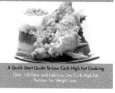
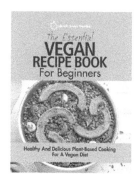
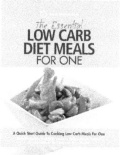
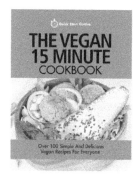
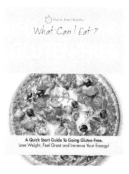

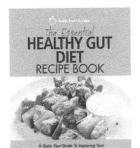

The Essential
HEALTHY GUT DIET
RECIPE BOOK

A Quick Start Guide to Improving Your Digestion, Health And Wellbeing

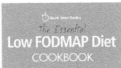

The Essential
Low FODMAP Diet
COOKBOOK

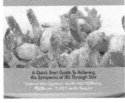

A Quick Start Guide To Relieving the Symptoms of IBS Through Diet

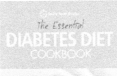

The Essential
DIABETES DIET
COOKBOOK

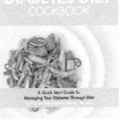

A Quick Start Guide To Managing Your Diabetes Through Diet

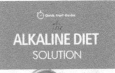

The
ALKALINE DIET
SOLUTION

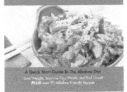

A Quick Start Guide To The Alkaline Diet

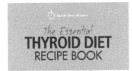

The Essential
THYROID DIET
RECIPE BOOK

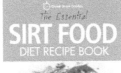

The Essential
SIRT FOOD
DIET RECIPE BOOK

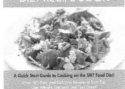

A Quick Start Guide to Cooking on the SIRT Food Diet

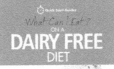

What Can I Eat?
ON A
DAIRY FREE
DIET

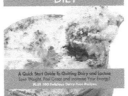

A Quick Start Guide To Quitting Dairy and Lactose

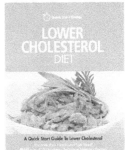

LOWER CHOLESTEROL
DIET

A Quick Start Guide To Lower Cholesterol

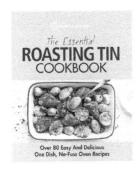

The Essential
ROASTING TIN
COOKBOOK

Over 80 Easy And Delicious One Dish, No-Fuss Oven Recipes

RECIPE JOURNAL

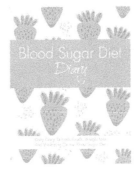

Blood Sugar Diet
Diary

Diabetes Diet
Diary

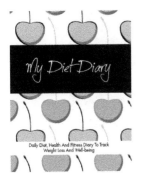

My Diet Diary

Daily Diet, Health And Fitness Diary To Track Weight Loss And Well-being

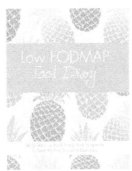

Low FODMAP
Food Diary

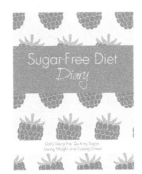

Sugar-Free Diet
Diary

Daily Diary For Quitting Sugar, Losing Weight and Feeling Great

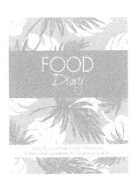

FOOD
Diary

You may also be interested in titles by
Pomegranate Journals

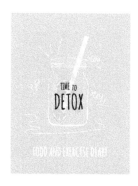

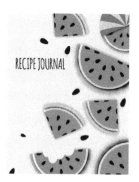
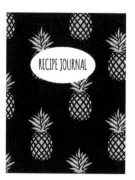
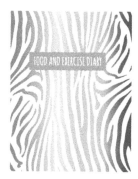
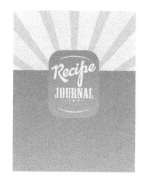
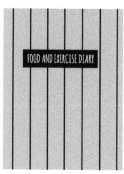
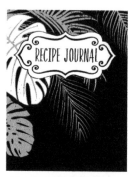

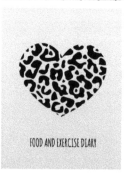
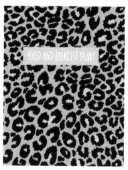
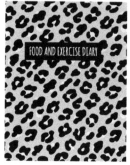

Lightning Source UK Ltd.
Milton Keynes UK
UKHW031848231019
352161UK00008B/137/P